# EVERYTHING TESTICULAR CANCER AND DIET

Comprehensive Guide To Germ Cell Tumours, Meal Plans, Foods To Eat And Avoid, Recipes, Nutritional Tips For Prevention And Recovery

**WALTON USELTON**

© 2024 [WALTON USELTON]

All rights reserved. No part of this book may be reproduced, distributed, or transmitted in any form or by any means, including photocopying, recording, or other electronic or mechanical methods, without the publisher's prior written permission, with the exception of brief quotations in critical reviews and certain other noncommercial uses permitted by copyright law.

# DISCLAIMER

The content in this book is based on the author's expertise and understanding of food and nutrition. The author is not linked or associated with any corporation, business, or person. This book is designed for informative purposes only and should not be interpreted as professional medical advice. Readers should get medical advice before making any changes to their diet or lifestyle. The author takes no responsibility or liability for any repercussions arising from the use of the information included in this book.

## Table of Contents

### INTRODUCTION ..... 13
- Understanding Testicular Cancer ..... 13
- Definition And Types Of Testicular Cancer ..... 14
- Risk Factors And Prevalence ..... 14
- The Importance Of Early Detection ..... 15
- The Role Of Diet In Prevention And Management ..... 16
- The Purpose Of This Book ..... 16

### CHAPTER ONE ..... 19
- Basics Of Nutrition ..... 19
- Importance Of A Balanced Diet ..... 19
- Nutrients Needed For Overall Health ..... 20
- Understanding Calories And Macronutrients ..... 21
- Importance Of Hydration ..... 22
- How Diet Affects Cancer Risk ..... 23

### CHAPTER TWO ..... 25
- Causes And Risks Of Testicular Cancer ..... 25
- Genetic Predisposition: Investigating The Role Of Genetics In Testicular Cancer ..... 25
- Environmental Factors: Navigating The Impact Of The Environment ..... 26

Lifestyle Choices And Habits: The Power Of Personal Decisions ..................................................... 27

Age And Ethnicity Considerations: Navigating Demographic Dynamics ............................................ 29

Other Medical Conditions And Their Relationship: Exploring Interconnected Health Dynamics ......................................................................... 30

## CHAPTER THREE ............................................................. 33

Dietary Guidelines For Testicular Cancer Prevention ....................................................................... 33

The Significance Of Fruits And Vegetables ........... 33

Whole Grains And Their Benefits .......................... 34

Lean Protein Sources ............................................. 36

Healthy Fats And Their Role .................................. 37

Limit Processed Foods And Sugary Beverages .. 39

## CHAPTER FOUR ................................................................ 41

Nutritional Support During Treatment ................ 41

Managing Side Effects With Diet .......................... 41

Adequate Caloric And Protein Intake ................... 42

Importance Of Hydration During Treatment .... 44

Foods That Relieve Nausea And Vomiting .......... 45

Adjusting Diet Based On Treatment Type .......... 47

## CHAPTER FIVE ... 49
### Supplements And Their Role ... 49
### Understanding Supplements ... 49
### Supplements Frequently Used During Cancer Treatment ... 50
#### 1. Vitamins and Minerals: ... 50
### Risks And Benefits Of Supplementation ... 52
#### 1. Potential Interactions: ... 52
#### 2. Safety Concerns: ... 52
#### 4. Cost Considerations: ... 53
#### 5. Nutritional Balance: ... 53
### Consultation With Healthcare Professionals ... 53
### Integrating Supplements And Diet ... 55
#### 1. Eating a Variety of Foods: ... 55
#### 4. Balanced Nutrient Intake: ... 56

## CHAPTER SIX ... 57
### Eat Well After Treatment ... 57
### Gradual Reintroduction Of Foods ... 57
### Creating A Sustainable Eating Plan ... 58
### Importance Of Regular Physical Activity ... 59
### Managing Long-Term Side Effects ... 61

Emotional Support And Wellbeing ........................ 62
CHAPTER SEVEN ................................................. 65
Developing Healthier Eating Habits ..................... 65
Mindful Eating Practices ........................................ 65
Meal Planning And Preparation Tips ................... 66
Portion Control Strategies ..................................... 68
Importance Of Maintaining A Regular Eating Schedule ................................................................... 69
Managing Appetites And Excesses ........................ 70
CHAPTER EIGHT ................................................. 73
Managing Specific Dietary Concerns .................... 73
Food Safety Throughout Treatment ..................... 73
Dealing With Taste Changes .................................. 75
Digestive Issues And Dietary Adjustments .......... 77
Coping With Dietary Restrictions ......................... 79
Seeking Professional Nutritional Counsel ........... 81
CHAPTER NINE ................................................... 83
Lifestyle Factors And Their Impact ...................... 83
The Importance Of Exercise And Physical Activity ..................................................................... 83
Stress Management Techniques ........................... 84

Quality Sleep And Its Role In Recovery ............... 87
Avoiding Tobacco And Excessive Alcohol ........... 89
Social Support And Community Engagement .... 90
CHAPTER TEN ................................................................ 93
Moving Forward: Long-Term Health And Wellness .................................................................. 93
Importance Of Regular Follow-Up Care ............... 93
Monitoring For Recurrence And Secondary Cancers ................................................................... 94
Healthy Lifestyle As A Preventive Measure ....... 96
Advocacy And Raising Awareness ........................ 97
Resources For Ongoing Support And Information ............................................................. 99
CONCLUSION ............................................................ 101
THE END ........................................................................ 103

## ABOUT THIS BOOK

"Testicular Cancer And Diet" is an excellent resource designed to provide persons with testicular cancer with extensive information and practical techniques centered on nutrition and lifestyle. From demystifying the complexities of testicular cancer to demonstrating the critical role of nutrition in prevention, care, and post-treatment recovery, this book is a beacon of hope and support.

The introduction portion provides readers with a firm basis, explaining the subtleties of testicular cancer, its numerous kinds, common risk factors, and the critical need for early identification. By clarifying the relationship between nutrition and testicular cancer, this book charts a clear path toward accepting dietary treatments as a preventative approach against this powerful illness.

The next chapters dig into the fundamentals of nutrition, emphasizing the significance of eating a well-balanced diet rich in important nutrients. Readers get insights into the relationship between food choices and cancer risk, allowing them to make educated decisions for their health. Furthermore, this book delves further into the causes and risk factors for testicular cancer, including genetic predispositions, environmental impacts, lifestyle decisions, and demographic concerns.

Chapter 3 is important to this book's concept since it outlines realistic dietary suggestions particularly designed for testicular cancer prevention. Readers are given practical techniques to strengthen their dietary defenses against cancer development and progression, with an emphasis on the importance of fruits, vegetables, whole grains, lean proteins, and healthy fats.

During the difficult road of treatment, Chapter 4 provides a lifeline of nutritional assistance, including techniques to reduce treatment-related side effects via individualized dietary treatments. Readers are led through the maze of therapy with practical and evidence-based dietary suggestions that include everything from nausea management to hydration and protein consumption.

Supplements become a main subject of discussion in Chapter 5 when readers learn about their possible advantages and hazards, as well as the need to contact healthcare specialists for personalized advice. Following therapy, Chapter 6 guides readers through the process of rebuilding food habits and regaining optimum health, emphasizing the symbiotic link between nutrition, physical exercise, and mental well-being.

Beyond food issues, This book delves into lifestyle aspects, highlighting the critical importance of exercise, stress management, adequate sleep, and social support in promoting overall recovery and long-term well-being.

This book acts as a reliable companion on the path to long-term health and vitality by advocating for frequent follow-up treatment, monitoring for recurrence, and cultivating an advocacy and awareness culture.

In short, "Testicular Cancer And Diet" goes beyond the bounds of traditional literature, encapsulating a comprehensive philosophy for empowerment, resistance, and well-being. It exemplifies the transformational power of information, empowering readers to handle the difficulties of testicular cancer with grace, courage, and unshakable optimism.

# INTRODUCTION

Testicular carcinoma is a kind of cancer that affects the testicles, which are part of the male reproductive system. It mostly affects young males, with the largest frequency happening among those aged 15 to 35. Understanding testicular cancer entails understanding its description, different kinds, risk factors, and the significance of early identification. Diet is important in both the prevention and treatment of this condition. In this book, we'll look at the role of nutrition in treating testicular cancer, offering practical advice and insights to help you make educated health decisions.

## Understanding Testicular Cancer

Testicular cancer is a disease that affects the testicles, which are part of the male reproductive system and produce sperm and testosterone. When aberrant cells begin to grow uncontrolled in the testicles, tumors develop, which may be malignant. There are two forms of testicular cancer: germ cell tumors and non-germ cell tumors. Germ cell tumors are the most prevalent form, accounting for over 95% of all occurrences.

## Definition And Types Of Testicular Cancer

Germ cell tumors arise from sperm-producing cells, but non-germ cell tumors form from other kinds of cells in the testicles, such as Leydig cells or Sertoli cells. Seminomas and non-seminomas are two types of germ cell tumors, each with its own set of features and therapeutic options. Seminomas often develop and spread more slowly than non-seminomas, although both forms need immediate medical attention and treatment.

## Risk Factors And Prevalence

Age, family history, an undecided testicle (cryptorchidism), a prior history of testicular cancer, and certain genetic diseases such as Klinefelter syndrome may all raise the chance of getting the disease. However, having one or more risk factors does not ensure the development of cancer, and those who do not have any risk factors may nonetheless acquire the disease. Testicular cancer is uncommon compared to other forms of cancer, yet it is the most prevalent malignancy among young men aged 15 to 35.

## The Importance Of Early Detection

Early identification of testicular cancer improves treatment results and enhances the likelihood of a full recovery. Regular self-examination of the testicles is critical for early detection since it helps men to recognize any anomalies, such as lumps or swelling, and seek medical assistance immediately. Routine clinical exams are also recommended by healthcare practitioners as part of preventative treatment, particularly for those who are at a greater risk owing to personal or family history.

# The Role Of Diet In Prevention And Management

While nutrition alone cannot prevent or cure testicular cancer, eating a balanced diet high in fruits, vegetables, whole grains, and lean meats may improve general health and well-being, perhaps lowering the chance of cancer. Antioxidant-rich foods like berries, tomatoes, and leafy greens can protect cells from free radical damage, possibly lowering the chance of developing cancer. Furthermore, eating vitamin D-rich foods like fatty fish, fortified dairy products, and eggs may help protect against some forms of cancer, including testicular cancer.

# The Purpose Of This Book

The goal of this book is to give complete information on testicular cancer, including its causes, risk factors, diagnosis, treatment choices, and preventative measures.

Understanding the illness and its related risks allows people to take proactive efforts to lower their risk, discover cancer early, and seek appropriate medical treatment. Furthermore, This book intends to provide readers with actionable ideas for preserving general health and well-being via lifestyle changes such as food choices and frequent exercise. Individuals with the necessary information and resources may make educated health choices and take charge of their testicular cancer prevention and treatment journey.

# CHAPTER ONE

## Basics Of Nutrition

## Importance Of A Balanced Diet

A well-balanced diet functions similarly to the gasoline that runs your body's engine. Just like a vehicle needs the proper combination of petrol, oil, and other fluids to operate effectively, your body requires a variety of nutrients to function properly. Carbohydrates, proteins, lipids, vitamins, and minerals are all essential for good health. A balanced diet ensures that you obtain all of the essential nutrients in the proper amounts, which helps to support body processes, maintain energy levels, and promote overall well-being.

A balanced diet should include a range of foods from various dietary categories. This includes lots of fruits and vegetables for vitamins, minerals, and fiber, as well as lean protein sources such as chicken, fish, beans, and nuts. Whole grains supply carbs for energy, and healthy fats found in avocados, olive oil, and nuts are required for cell function and hormone synthesis.

## Nutrients Needed For Overall Health

Various nutrients play important roles in general health, and each performs a unique set of tasks inside the body. Calcium, for example, is necessary for bone health; iron aids in the transportation of oxygen in the blood; and vitamin C supports the immune system. Consuming a varied selection of meals ensures that your body receives all of the critical nutrients it needs to function.

In addition to vitamins and minerals, other vital nutrients include antioxidants, which help protect cells from free radical damage, and fiber, which promotes digestion and may reduce the risk of certain illnesses. By prioritizing nutrient-dense foods in your diet, you can give your body the resources it needs to be healthy and operate properly.

## Understanding Calories And Macronutrients

Calories are units of energy derived from the food and drinks we eat. Your daily calorie need is determined by a variety of variables, including your age, gender, weight, height, and degree of exercise. taking more calories than your body requires may cause weight growth while taking fewer calories can cause weight reduction.

Macronutrients, or macros for short, are the three major calorie-containing components of food: carbs, proteins, and fat. Carbohydrates are the body's principal source of energy, whereas proteins are necessary for tissue growth and repair, and lipids contribute to cell structure and hormone synthesis. Balancing your macronutrient consumption is essential for maintaining a balanced diet and meeting your body's demands.

## Importance Of Hydration

Proper hydration is critical for overall health and well-being. Water makes up a large component of our bodies and is engaged in a variety of physiological functions such as temperature regulation, nutrition delivery, and waste removal. Dehydration may cause weariness, dizziness, and other symptoms, so drink plenty of fluids throughout the day to keep well hydrated.

In addition to water, herbal teas, and low-fat milk may help you stay hydrated throughout the day. Fruits and vegetables are also rich in water content, making them hydrating dietary options. Drink water often throughout the day, particularly before, during, and after activity, to restore fluids lost via perspiration and avoid dehydration.

## How Diet Affects Cancer Risk

Diet has a substantial impact on cancer risk, with various foods and dietary patterns being linked to either an increased or reduced possibility of acquiring cancer. A diet rich in processed meats, sugary beverages, and refined carbs has been associated with an increased risk of malignancies such as colorectal, breast, and pancreatic.

On the other side, a diet high in fruits, vegetables, whole grains, and lean meats has been linked to a decreased risk of cancer. These foods include a range of vitamins, minerals, antioxidants, and phytochemicals that have been demonstrated to have cancer-preventing properties. Adopting a balanced eating pattern and selecting nutritious food choices may lower your risk of cancer while also improving your general health and well-being.

# CHAPTER TWO

## Causes And Risks Of Testicular Cancer

## Genetic Predisposition: Investigating The Role Of Genetics In Testicular Cancer

Understanding the hereditary propensity for testicular cancer is critical. It's like figuring out a hard puzzle. Genes influence our vulnerability to a variety of illnesses, including testicular cancer.

Imagine your DNA as a blueprint that governs how your body works and responds to various stimuli. Some people may inherit genetic alterations that make them susceptible to testicular cancer. These mutations may disrupt the normal control of cell growth and division, resulting in the formation of malignant tumors in the testicles.

Specific genetic abnormalities, such as changes in genes like BRCA1 and BRCA2, have been related to an increased risk of testicular cancer in males. Understanding your genetic composition via genetic testing may give useful insights into your risk profile, guiding personalized screening and preventative plans.

## Environmental Factors: Navigating The Impact Of The Environment

The environment plays an important part in the complex web of elements that contribute to testicular cancer. Consider the environment to be a dynamic landscape full of variables that may either encourage or prevent cancer growth.

Exposure to some environmental contaminants, chemicals, and pollutants has been linked to testicular cancer. For example, industrial pollutants such as phthalates, insecticides, and solvents have been linked to an increased chance of getting testicular cancer. Furthermore, radiation exposure, whether from medical imaging techniques or workplace dangers, might enhance vulnerability to this illness.

Understanding the environmental elements at play enables people to make educated choices that reduce exposure and risk. Taking proactive actions to decrease environmental exposures, such as adopting eco-friendly behaviors or campaigning for workplace safety measures, may be an effective method for preventing testicular cancer.

## Lifestyle Choices And Habits: The Power Of Personal Decisions

Our lifestyle choices and behaviors have a substantial impact on our health outcomes, including the likelihood of acquiring testicular cancer. Consider how our everyday choices shape our health trajectory, similar to negotiating a meandering path to well-being.

Maintaining a healthy lifestyle, which includes regular exercise, a balanced diet, and avoiding dangerous behaviors such as smoking and excessive alcohol use, may dramatically reduce the chance of developing testicular cancer. Consuming antioxidant-rich foods, such as fruits, vegetables, and whole grains, might help neutralize damaging free radicals and improve general cellular health.

Furthermore, maintaining a healthy body weight and avoiding obesity might help prevent testicular cancer. Obesity is more than a cosmetic issue; it is a complicated metabolic disease that may exacerbate inflammation and hormone imbalances, producing an environment susceptible to cancer development.

Individuals may improve their chances of avoiding testicular cancer by making purposeful decisions to prioritize their health and well-being. It's about empowering yourself to take charge of your health and develop habits that promote longevity and vitality.

## Age And Ethnicity Considerations: Navigating Demographic Dynamics

Age and ethnicity are major demographic factors that might affect the risk of testicular cancer. Consider them as glasses through which we might observe the landscape of cancer epidemiology, providing insights into the patterns and trends that define our knowledge of the illness.

Testicular cancer typically affects young males, with the highest incidence happening between the ages of 15 and 40. This demographic skew emphasizes the necessity of early identification and awareness campaigns for young males who may be at risk.

Furthermore, ethnicity influences susceptibility to testicular cancer, with some racial and ethnic groupings having greater incidence rates than others. For example, Caucasian males are more likely to acquire testicular cancer than men of African or Asian heritage. Understanding these demographic differences may help inspire focused screening and preventative initiatives for certain groups.

Recognizing the relationship between age, ethnicity, and testicular cancer risk allows healthcare professionals and people to take proactive actions to diagnose and reduce the burden of this illness across varied demographic groups.

## Other Medical Conditions And Their Relationship: Exploring Interconnected Health Dynamics

Human health is a complicated network of interconnected medical disorders. Understanding the link between testicular cancer and other medical disorders provides useful insights into overall health management techniques.

Certain medical problems and therapies may influence testicular cancer risk or diagnosis. Individuals with undecided testicles (cryptorchidism) have a higher chance of acquiring testicular cancer later in life. Furthermore, having a history of testicular cancer in one testicle doubles the likelihood of acquiring cancer in the other.

Furthermore, the treatment of other malignancies, such as Hodgkin lymphoma, sometimes includes radiation therapy or chemotherapy, which may impair testicular function and raise the risk of recurrent testicular cancer. Healthcare practitioners must consider these interrelated health dynamics when developing treatment regimens and monitoring techniques for individuals with multiple medical disorders.

Healthcare practitioners may optimize patient care and enhance outcomes throughout the cancer prevention, diagnosis, and treatment continuum by using a holistic approach to health management that takes into account the interaction between testicular cancer and other medical disorders.

# CHAPTER THREE

## Dietary Guidelines For Testicular Cancer Prevention

## The Significance Of Fruits And Vegetables

Fruits and vegetables are like diet superheroes when it comes to avoiding testicular cancer. They are high in critical vitamins, minerals, and antioxidants, and they work hard to boost your immune system and combat cancer-causing toxins. Consider them your body's defense team, swooping in to neutralize dangerous free radicals and keep your cells healthy.

However, it is important to consider diversity as well as quantity. Each fruit and vegetable provides a distinct collection of nutrients. For example, leafy greens like spinach and kale are high in folate, a B vitamin that may help reduce the risk of some malignancies, including testicular cancer. Meanwhile, brightly colored foods such as berries and citrus fruits are high in vitamin C, another potent antioxidant that promotes immune function and aids in cell repair.

The goal is to load your plate with a variety of colors and aim for at least five servings of fruits and vegetables every day. Every mouthful, whether you're crunching carrots, slicing strawberries, or making a kale smoothie, takes you closer to maximum health and cancer prevention.

## Whole Grains And Their Benefits

When it comes to preventing testicular cancer, whole grains are the diet's hidden heroes. Whole grains, as opposed to processed grains, are rich in fiber and nutrients due to the bran, germ, and endosperm. This means they not only keep you feeling fuller for longer, but they also deliver a consistent stream of energy and critical nutrients to help you stay healthy.

But arguably their most significant achievement is their ability to lower the risk of certain diseases, particularly testicular cancer. Whole grains, with their high fiber content, help keep your digestive system operating smoothly, minimizing the amount of time that possible carcinogens come into touch with your intestinal walls. Furthermore, they contain antioxidants and other phytochemicals that aid in the fight against inflammation and oxidative stress, both of which are major contributors to cancer formation.

So, what precisely constitutes a whole grain? Consider more than just whole wheat bread; oats, quinoa, brown rice, barley, and buckwheat are just a few examples of whole grains that may be readily introduced into your diet. Whether you're beginning your day with a healthy bowl of muesli or replacing white rice with brown, switching to whole grains is a little adjustment that may have a significant impact on your cancer prevention goals.

## Lean Protein Sources

Protein is necessary for the development and repair of tissues in your body, but not all sources are created equal, particularly when it comes to testicular cancer prevention. While red and processed meats have been linked to an increased risk of various malignancies, including testicular cancer, switching to lean protein sources may help protect your health.

So, what precisely is considered a lean protein? Think about chicken, fish, beans, lentils, tofu, and low-fat dairy items. These selections are not only lower in saturated fat and cholesterol than red meat, but they also include additional nutrients that promote general health.

Fish, in particular, deserve special attention due to its high omega-3 fatty acid concentration. According to studies, omega-3s may help decrease inflammation and lessen the risk of some malignancies, making fish a good option for testicular cancer prevention. To enjoy the most advantages, consume fatty fish such as salmon, mackerel, and sardines at least twice a week.

Instead of frying, prepare lean meats using healthier ways such as grilling, baking, steaming, or sautéing. Also, remember to combine your protein sources with lots of fruits, veggies, and whole grains to produce a well-balanced meal that promotes general health and cancer prevention.

## Healthy Fats And Their Role

Unlike common assumptions, not all fats are harmful to you. In truth, healthy fats are essential for maintaining good health and may even lower the risk of some diseases, such as testicular cancer. The idea is to choose the proper fats and consume them in moderation.

When it comes to preventing testicular cancer, monounsaturated and polyunsaturated fats shine brightest. These fats, which may be found in nuts, seeds, avocados, and fatty fish, have been proven to decrease inflammation, enhance heart health, and even lessen the chance of cancer formation.

Meanwhile, saturated and trans fats, which are present in red and processed meats, fried meals, and many processed snacks, should be reduced or avoided entirely. When ingested in excess, these fats may elevate cholesterol levels and increase the risk of heart disease, as well as contribute to inflammation and cancer formation.

When adding healthy fats to your diet, strive for balance and moderation. Sprinkle a handful of almonds over your morning muesli, sprinkle olive oil over your salad, or spread avocado over whole-grain toast for a filling and cancer-fighting snack. Making wise decisions and prioritizing healthy fats will improve your overall health while also lowering your chance of testicular cancer.

# Limit Processed Foods And Sugary Beverages

When it comes to preventing testicular cancer, what you don't consume is as essential as what you do. Processed foods and sugary drinks are renowned for containing high quantities of sugar, salt, bad fats, and chemical additives, all of which have been related to an increased risk of cancer.

Excess sugar intake, in particular, has been linked to inflammation, insulin resistance, and obesity—all of which are risk factors for testicular cancer. Sugary beverages, including soda, fruit juices, and energy drinks, are some of the most common sources of hidden sugars in the diet, so limit your consumption and instead choose water, herbal tea, or infused water.

Similarly, processed meats such as hot dogs, bacon, and deli meats sometimes include preservatives and additives that raise the risk of cancer. Reducing your consumption of these foods and switching to whole, less processed alternatives may help decrease your cancer risk and enhance your general health.

You may minimize your risk of testicular cancer and promote optimum health for years to come by prioritizing full, nutrient-dense foods such as fruits, vegetables, whole grains, lean proteins, and healthy fats, as well as reducing your consumption of processed foods and sugary drinks.

# CHAPTER FOUR

## Nutritional Support During Treatment

## Managing Side Effects With Diet

Dietary management of side effects during testicular cancer therapy is critical to overall well-being. Various treatment procedures, including chemotherapy, radiation therapy, and surgery, may cause unpleasant side effects such as nausea, vomiting, exhaustion, and loss of appetite. However, with proper nutritional assistance, these adverse effects may be reduced, enabling patients to endure therapy and keep their vigor.

Maintaining a proper calorie and protein intake is an important part of controlling adverse effects. Cancer therapies may raise the body's energy requirements, so it's critical to consume enough calories to avoid weight loss and muscle withering. Protein is especially crucial for tissue repair and immunological function, both of which might be impaired during therapy. Protein-rich meals such as lean meats, poultry, fish, eggs, dairy products, beans, and nuts may assist fulfill your higher protein requirements.

Another important aspect is hydration. Many cancer therapies may induce dehydration, either directly or indirectly, due to side effects such as vomiting and diarrhea. Staying hydrated is vital for good physical function and overall wellness. Drinking lots of fluids, such as water, herbal teas, broth, and electrolyte-replacement beverages, may help avoid dehydration and relieve symptoms like dry mouth and weariness.

## Adequate Caloric And Protein Intake

Individuals receiving testicular cancer therapy must ensure they consume a proper quantity of calories and protein. Cancer therapies may raise the body's energy needs, therefore it's critical to consume enough calories to maintain weight and energy levels. Furthermore, proper protein consumption is critical for immunological function, muscle preservation, and tissue regeneration.

To satisfy calorie requirements, eat nutrient-dense meals that provide important vitamins, minerals, and antioxidants. Include a variety of fruits, vegetables, whole grains, lean meats, and healthy fats in your diet to promote a well-balanced nutritional profile. Consuming calorie-dense foods such as nuts, seeds, avocados, and oils may also aid increase calorie consumption without increasing meal size.

Protein-rich foods should be included in all meals and snacks to aid with muscle regeneration and immunological function. Include protein in each meal, such as lean meats, poultry, fish, eggs, dairy products, legumes, tofu, and tempeh. If you are concerned about your hunger, eating smaller, more frequent meals and snacks throughout the day will help you get enough calories and protein without overloading your digestive system.

## Importance Of Hydration During Treatment

Individuals receiving testicular cancer therapy must be well-hydrated. Cancer therapies, such as chemotherapy and radiation therapy, may raise the risk of dehydration owing to side effects such as vomiting, diarrhea, and reduced appetite. Dehydration may aggravate other treatment-related adverse effects, jeopardizing general health and well-being.

To keep properly hydrated, drink enough fluids throughout the day, even if you don't feel thirsty. Water is the greatest option for hydration, although herbal teas, clear broths, and electrolyte-replenishment beverages may also help. Avoid sugary drinks and caffeine, since these may cause dehydration and exacerbate symptoms such as nausea and exhaustion.

In addition to drinking water, eating hydrating meals may help you stay hydrated. Fruits and vegetables with high water content, such as watermelon, oranges, and strawberries, may help you stay hydrated while also supplying critical vitamins, minerals, and antioxidants.

## Foods That Relieve Nausea And Vomiting

Cancer treatments such as chemotherapy and radiation therapy can cause nausea and vomiting. These symptoms may be upsetting, affecting both appetite and quality of life. Certain dietary techniques, on the other hand, may help decrease nausea and vomiting, making therapy more bearable and allowing for enough nourishment.

Choosing bland, readily digested meals might help calm the stomach and prevent nausea. Examples include crackers, bread, rice, bananas, applesauce, and plain yogurt. Avoiding oily, spicy, or highly flavored meals may also assist in alleviating nausea and avoiding vomiting.

Ginger has long been used as a natural cure for nausea, and it may be ingested in a variety of forms such as ginger tea, ginger ale, and ginger candy. Drinking peppermint tea or sucking on peppermint candies may also assist with nausea and digestion.

Eating smaller, more frequent meals throughout the day may help reduce nausea caused by an empty stomach. It is important to listen to your body and eat when you are hungry, even if it is outside of your usual mealtimes.

# Adjusting Diet Based On Treatment Type

Dietary guidelines and concerns for testicular cancer patients might be influenced by their treatment type. For example, people receiving chemotherapy may have changes in taste and appetite, making it difficult to eat specific meals. In contrast, patients receiving radiation treatment may encounter localized adverse effects such as mouth sores or trouble swallowing, which might influence meal choices.

Even if your appetite is suppressed, it is critical to keep hydrated and consume enough calories and protein while receiving chemotherapy. Choosing appetizing and easy-to-digest meals may help avoid malnutrition and promote general health.

Individuals suffering from mouth sores or trouble swallowing as a result of radiation treatment might find relief in soft, moist meals that are simple to chew and swallow. It is also suggested that you avoid spicy, acidic, or rough-textured meals that might irritate your tongue or throat.

In rare circumstances, dietary supplements or nutritional smoothies may be prescribed to guarantee proper nutrient intake, particularly if eating solid meals is difficult. Consulting with a certified dietitian or healthcare professional may assist in tailoring dietary advice to individual requirements and preferences during the treatment process.

# CHAPTER FIVE

## Supplements And Their Role

## Understanding Supplements

Supplements are items that include one or more nutritional elements and are designed to augment a person's diet. They are available in numerous forms, including tablets, capsules, powders, and liquids. These items might include vitamins, minerals, herbs, amino acids, enzymes, or other ingredients.

Supplements may help persons undergoing cancer treatment maintain their general health and well-being. However, it is critical to recognize that supplements are intended to augment, not replace, a healthy diet. To get the most advantages, they should be utilized in combination with good eating habits.

When contemplating supplements, it is important to be knowledgeable about their components, potential interactions with drugs, and adverse effects. Consulting with a healthcare expert, such as a doctor or dietician, may assist verify that the supplements selected are safe and suitable for your specific requirements.

## Supplements Frequently Used During Cancer Treatment

Several supplements are regularly taken by cancer patients to assist control of symptoms and improve overall health. This may include:

1. **Vitamins and Minerals:** Certain vitamins and minerals, such as vitamin D, vitamin B12, calcium, and zinc, may be prescribed to aid with nutritional deficits or immunological function.

2. Herbal supplements, such as ginger, turmeric, and green tea extract, are often utilized for their anti-inflammatory and antioxidant qualities. They may

help to reduce nausea, inflammation, and oxidative stress caused by cancer therapy.

3. Probiotics are helpful bacteria that may help keep gut flora in balance, which is necessary for digestion and immunological function. They may also assist with gastrointestinal side effects from cancer therapy, such as diarrhea and constipation.

4. Fish oil supplements include omega-3 fatty acids, which are believed to have anti-inflammatory qualities. During cancer therapy, they may help decrease inflammation, increase appetite, and promote overall heart health.

5. Antioxidants: Supplements containing antioxidants such as vitamin C, vitamin E, and selenium may help protect cells against free radical damage, which is a consequence of normal cell metabolism that may contribute to cancer growth and progression.

# Risks And Benefits Of Supplementation

While supplements may provide potential advantages, several concerns should be carefully considered:

**1. Potential Interactions:** Some supplements may interact with drugs or other supplements, reducing their effectiveness or producing side effects. To prevent hazardous interactions, report any supplements used to healthcare practitioners.

**2. Safety Concerns:** Certain supplements may be dangerous, particularly when used in large dosages or over long periods. For example, taking too much vitamin E or beta-carotene supplements may raise your chance of developing some malignancies.

3. The quality and purity of supplements might vary greatly across brands and manufacturers. Selecting recognized brands that have undergone third-party

testing for quality and purity may help reduce the danger of contamination or adulteration.

**4. Cost Considerations:** Supplements may be expensive, particularly if used regularly over time. It is critical to balance the potential advantages against the financial burden and to investigate more economical options wherever available.

**5. Nutritional Balance:** Relying too heavily on supplements may result in an imbalance in nutrient intake, diminishing the necessity of a well-rounded diet. It is critical to prioritize entire meals and dietary sources of nutrients wherever available.

## Consultation With Healthcare Professionals

Before beginning any supplement program, contact a healthcare expert, such as a doctor or dietician. They may provide personalized suggestions based on an individual's health situation, nutritional requirements, and treatment objectives.

## During consultations, healthcare practitioners can:

• Evaluate current food consumption and nutritional status to identify shortfalls or opportunities for improvement.

• Check medical history and current medicines for any possible interactions or contraindications.

• Advise on choosing suitable supplements, including dose, frequency, and duration of usage.

• Monitor and adapt supplement regimen depending on individual reaction and treatment results.

Working together with healthcare providers may help patients guarantee the safe and successful use of supplements to enhance their overall health and well-being throughout cancer treatment.

# Integrating Supplements And Diet

Supplements should be considered as one component of a more holistic approach to nutrition and well-being. While they may help, they should not be used instead of a nutritious diet rich in fruits, vegetables, whole grains, lean meats, and healthy fats.

## Integrating supplements with the diet entails:

1. **Eating a Variety of Foods:** Try to include a variety of nutrient-dense foods into your diet to guarantee optimal consumption of key vitamins, minerals, and other nutrients.

2. Prioritise entire foods as the major source of nutrients, such as fruits, vegetables, whole grains, legumes, nuts, seeds, and lean proteins.

3. Strategic supplementation entails filling nutritional shortfalls or addressing specific problems discovered via collaboration with healthcare practitioners.

4. **Balanced Nutrient Intake:** To maintain maximum health and well-being, avoid excessive supplementing and aim for a balanced intake of nutrients from both food and supplement sources.

Individuals may optimize their nutritional intake and improve general well-being before and after cancer treatment by carefully using supplements in combination with a nutritious diet.

# CHAPTER SIX

## Eat Well After Treatment

## Gradual Reintroduction Of Foods

After receiving treatment for testicular cancer, it is important to pay attention to your nutrition to assist your recovery and general health. One important part is to gradually reintroduce foods into your diet. During therapy, your body may have changed its appetite, digestion, and tolerance to specific meals. As a result, carefully reintroducing foods might help you detect any sensitivities or intolerances that may have arisen during therapy.

Begin by reintroducing meals that are readily digested, including cooked vegetables, lean meats, and whole grains. These meals include important nutrients without overpowering your digestive system.

As your tolerance grows, you may gradually reintroduce additional foods including dairy, fruits, and raw vegetables.

Listen to your body and be aware of any symptoms or pain that occur after eating specific meals. If you have any negative effects, such as bloating, gas, or nausea, try removing the meal from your diet briefly and returning it later. Keep a food journal to monitor your symptoms and uncover trends.

## Creating A Sustainable Eating Plan

Developing a sustainable food plan is critical for long-term health and well-being after testicular cancer treatment. A well-balanced diet rich in nutrient-dense foods may boost your immune system, improve healing, and minimize the chance of cancer recurrence.

Include a mix of fruits, vegetables, whole grains, lean meats, and healthy fats in your meals. Fill half of your plate with fruits and vegetables, a quarter with healthy grains, and the remaining quarter with lean meats like fish, chicken, tofu, or lentils. Choose whole foods over processed foods wherever feasible to increase nutritional intake while reducing added sugars, salt, and harmful fats.

Staying hydrated is also crucial, so drink lots of water throughout the day. Water promotes adequate hydration, aids digestion, and eliminates toxins from the body. Limit your consumption of sugary drinks and alcohol, since they may cause dehydration and have a bad influence on your health.

## Importance Of Regular Physical Activity

In addition to eating a balanced diet, frequent physical exercise is critical for general health and well-being during testicular cancer therapy. Exercise may increase strength, endurance, flexibility, and mood while also lowering the risk of other chronic conditions.

Begin with low-impact exercises like walking, swimming, or cycling, then gradually increase the intensity and duration as your strength and stamina improve. The American Cancer Society recommends at least 150 minutes of moderate-intensity exercise or 75 minutes of vigorous-intensity activity every week.

Include a range of activities in your daily routine to keep things fresh and avoid boredom or burnout. Consider taking a fitness class, trying out a new activity, or combining strength training routines to increase muscle mass and general fitness. Remember to listen to your body and adjust your workout regimen accordingly to suit any physical restrictions or obstacles.

# Managing Long-Term Side Effects

While the early negative effects of testicular cancer therapy may fade with time, some people may develop long-term side effects that need continuous care. Fatigue, neuropathy, hormone abnormalities, and changes in bowel or bladder function are all possibilities.

It's critical to collaborate with your healthcare team to address any remaining side effects and create a complete treatment strategy. Medication, physical therapy, dietary alterations, or lifestyle changes may all be used to assist reduce symptoms and enhance the quality of life.

Incorporating stress-relieving activities like mindfulness meditation, yoga, or deep breathing techniques may also help control long-term negative effects and maintain mental health. Furthermore, attending a support group or seeking individual counseling may give important emotional support and encouragement during this time.

## Emotional Support And Wellbeing

Emotional support and well-being are critical components of the healing process after testicular cancer therapy. Coping with a cancer diagnosis and treatment may be emotionally tough, so it's important to prioritize self-care and seek help when necessary.

Maintain contact with friends, family, and loved ones who can provide emotional support and encouragement during your healing process. Don't be afraid to communicate your emotions and seek assistance when necessary. Joining a support group or seeking counseling or therapy may also give important emotional support and coping methods.

Spending time in nature, participating in hobbies or artistic interests, and practicing mindfulness and meditation are all examples of self-care activities that promote relaxation and stress alleviation. Remember to be patient with yourself and give yourself time to recover, both physically and emotionally.

You may help your recovery and survival following testicular cancer treatment by concentrating on progressive food reintroduction, creating a sustainable nutrition plan, prioritizing regular physical exercise, controlling long-term side effects, and seeking mental support and well-being.

# CHAPTER SEVEN

## Developing Healthier Eating Habits

### Mindful Eating Practices

Mindful eating entails being present and completely involved in the act of eating. It entails paying attention to food's sensory sensations, such as taste, texture, and scent, as well as your body's hunger and fullness signals. This practice may help you build a healthy connection with food and make more informed decisions about what and how much to consume.

Slowing down and enjoying each meal is one method to practice mindful eating. Instead of hurrying through your meal, chew carefully and enjoy the flavors and sensations. This might help you feel more fulfilled and avoid overeating.

Another part of mindful eating is being aware of your body's hunger and fullness cues. Before you begin eating, check in with yourself to determine how hungry you are. During the meal, pay attention to how your body feels and stop eating when you begin to feel content, rather than waiting until you're too full.

It is also beneficial to limit distractions when eating, such as watching TV or going through your phone. By concentrating entirely on the process of eating, you may better understand your body's signals and appreciate your meal more thoroughly.

## Meal Planning And Preparation Tips

Meal planning is an important part of a healthy diet since it helps you to make informed decisions about what you eat and ensures that you have nutritious meals accessible. To begin meal planning, set aside some time each week to plan out your meals and create a shopping list.

When preparing your meals, strive for a variety of nutrients, such as lean proteins, whole grains, fruits, and vegetables. Try to incorporate a variety of foods to keep your meals interesting and to guarantee that you're receiving all of the nutrients your body requires.

After you've planned your meals, set aside some time to prepare as much as possible ahead of time. This might include cutting vegetables, preparing grains, or marinating meats. By performing some of the prep work ahead of time, you may save time and worry throughout the week.

When it comes to dinner preparation, keep things simple and stick to basic, healthful meals. Look for recipes with few ingredients and preparation time, or try batch-cooking bigger amounts of food to divide up and freeze for later.

# Portion Control Strategies

Portion management is essential for keeping a healthy weight and avoiding overeating. Using smaller dishes and bowls is an excellent way to limit portion sizes. According to research, individuals eat more when presented with bigger servings, therefore utilizing smaller plates might help you naturally eat less.

Another important approach is to consider serving sizes and suggested portion amounts. Many packaged goods have information on serving sizes on the nutrition label, but it may also be beneficial to get acquainted with typical portion sizes for various kinds of meals.

Visual cues may also be useful for estimating portion sizes. For example, a portion of meat or fish is normally the size of a deck of cards, but a serving of pasta or rice is around the size of a tennis ball.

Visualizing these servings allows you to better judge how much you should consume.

Finally, try to eat slowly and carefully, paying close attention to your body's hunger and fullness signals. Eating slowly allows your body to recognize sensations of fullness, which may assist avoid overeating.

## Importance Of Maintaining A Regular Eating Schedule

Maintaining a regular meal schedule is essential for maintaining consistent energy levels throughout the day and avoiding excessive hunger, which may lead to overeating. Aim to eat every 3-4 hours to keep your metabolism working normally and prevent blood sugar spikes and crashes.

Planning your meals and snacks ahead of time might help you keep to a regular eating pattern. This may assist you avoid missing meals or turning to harmful convenience foods when you're hungry.

It's also vital to pay attention to your body's hunger and fullness signals and eat when you're hungry, rather than out of habit or boredom. Tuning into your body's cues allows you to better control your eating habits and prevent unneeded snacking.

If you're hungry in between meals, look for nutritious snacks like fresh fruit, almonds, or yogurt to keep you full until your next meal. Avoiding prolonged hunger might assist avoid overeating later on.

## Managing Appetites And Excesses

Cravings are a normal part of life, but learning to control them may help you eat a healthier diet. One approach to coping with cravings is to uncover the root reason.

Are you seeking something sweet because you're tired or worried, or because you're really hungry? Understanding the underlying reason for your cravings allows you to handle them more effectively and healthily.

Another useful approach is to look for healthier alternatives to your favorite decadent dishes. For example, if you want something sweet, grab a piece of fruit or a modest dish of dark chocolate rather than a sugary dessert. Similarly, if you want something salty, choose air-popped popcorn or whole-grain crackers instead of chips.

It's also crucial to consume your favorite delicacies in moderation. Rather than fully denying yourself, allow yourself to indulge in little amounts of your favorite foods on occasion. You may fulfill your desires without jeopardizing your healthy eating habits by indulging in these delicacies in moderation and with mindfulness.

# CHAPTER EIGHT

## Managing Specific Dietary Concerns

## Food Safety Throughout Treatment

Keeping food safe during cancer treatment is critical to preserving general health and avoiding infections. Chemotherapy and radiation treatment impairs the immune system, rendering patients more vulnerable to food-borne diseases. As a result, it is essential to implement certain strategies to reduce the danger of contamination.

First, always properly wash your hands before handling food. This easy action may help prevent hazardous germs from being transferred to food. Furthermore, make sure that all fruits and vegetables are thoroughly cleaned under running water, even if they have peels that you do not consume.

When cooking meals, it is best to properly prepare dishes, particularly meat, poultry, and shellfish. Use a food thermometer to verify that meats achieve the required interior temperature to destroy any germs. Leftovers should be refrigerated and used within a few days to avoid spoiling.

Furthermore, avoid unpasteurized dairy products and uncooked eggs, since they might contain hazardous germs such as Salmonella. To reduce the risk of foodborne disease, use pasteurized dairy and cooked eggs.

Finally, be aware of cross-contamination in the kitchen. To minimize cross-contamination, keep raw meat, poultry, and shellfish on separate cutting surfaces and utensils. To maintain a sanitary cooking environment, sanitize kitchen surfaces regularly.

Cancer patients may lower their chances of contracting foodborne infections and improve their overall health by adhering to certain food safety standards during treatment.

## Dealing With Taste Changes

Chemotherapy and radiation treatment may often induce taste alterations, resulting in a reduced appetite or aversion to particular meals. Dealing with these flavor changes requires ingenuity and agility in meal planning.

One method is to try various flavors and textures to see what appeals to your taste. For example, if you notice that particular dishes taste bland or metallic, consider adding herbs, spices, or citrus flavors to improve the flavor. Sauces, marinades, and condiments may also help disguise disagreeable flavors.

Consider altering the temperature of meals to observe how they alter their flavor. Some people may prefer cold or room-temperature cuisine over hot ones.

Similarly, tasting foods at various stages of ripeness or cooking may result in diverse flavor profiles.

To properly prevent taste alterations, you must also keep hydrated and practice good dental hygiene. Drinking enough water throughout the day may help clean the palate and avoid dry mouth, which can worsen taste changes. Furthermore, proper dental hygiene, such as frequent brushing and flossing, might enhance flavor perception.

Finally, if you notice any taste changes, please notify your healthcare staff. They may provide further advice or prescribe drugs to relieve discomfort and enhance appetite.

Cancer patients may deal with taste changes and retain appropriate nutrition after treatment by trying new flavors, keeping hydrated, and maintaining excellent mouth hygiene.

# Digestive Issues And Dietary Adjustments

Cancer therapy often causes digestive problems such as nausea, vomiting, diarrhea, and constipation. These symptoms have a substantial influence on a patient's quality of life and nutritional intake. However, some dietary and lifestyle modifications may help control digestive difficulties more successfully.

Individuals suffering from nausea and vomiting should consume modest, regular meals throughout the day rather than big, heavy meals. Choose bland, easy-to-digest items like crackers, bread, rice, bananas, and applesauce. Avoid meals that are hot, fatty, or highly seasoned, since they might worsen nausea.

Similarly, persons experiencing diarrhea should consume low-fiber meals that are soothing to the digestive tract.

This contains white rice, boiled potatoes, skinless vegetables, and lean meats such as chicken or fish. Stay hydrated by consuming lots of fluids, but avoid caffeinated or carbonated drinks, which may worsen diarrhea.

Constipation, on the other hand, may be relieved by eating more fiber-rich foods such as whole grains, fruits, and vegetables. To promote bowel regularity, drink lots of water and exercise regularly.

Consider maintaining a food journal to monitor symptoms and discover possible trigger foods that might exacerbate digestive problems. This might help you modify your diet to meet your specific requirements and interests.

If digestive problems continue or worsen, speak with a doctor about personalized dietary suggestions or medicines to help manage symptoms successfully.

Cancer patients may enhance their overall well-being while undergoing treatment by implementing dietary and lifestyle modifications.

## Coping With Dietary Restrictions

Some cancer therapies may include dietary restrictions to improve efficacy or control adverse effects. Adhering to these limits might be difficult, but with careful planning and imagination, you can maintain a healthy and pleasant diet.

A low-sodium diet is a frequent dietary restriction that may be prescribed for people with certain forms of cancer or cardiovascular disease. Limit your consumption of processed and packaged foods, which are generally rich in sodium. Instead, choose fresh or less processed meals, and season dishes with herbs, spices, or citrus juice.

Another dietary limitation is a low-fiber diet, which may be recommended to treat digestive problems including diarrhea or bowel blockage. This usually means avoiding high-fiber foods like whole grains, raw fruits and vegetables, nuts, and seeds. Instead, concentrate on low-fiber, easy-to-digest choices.

Individuals receiving some cancer therapies may also need to restrict their consumption of key nutrients such as vitamin K, which might impair drug efficiency. In such circumstances, consult a qualified dietitian to devise a meal plan that satisfies nutritional requirements while sticking to dietary limitations.

It is critical to speak freely with healthcare practitioners and obtain expert dietary advice to ensure that dietary restrictions are followed safely and successfully. With appropriate preparation and assistance, cancer patients may negotiate food limitations while maintaining optimum nutrition and well-being during treatment.

# Seeking Professional Nutritional Counsel

Navigating the complexity of food and nutrition during cancer treatment may be difficult, but obtaining expert dietary advice can give vital help and support. Registered dietitians specialize in creating personalized nutrition regimens based on individual requirements and treatment objectives.

A certified dietitian may evaluate eating patterns, address particular nutritional problems, and provide practical solutions for improving nutrition throughout cancer treatment. They may also help you manage side effects including taste changes, intestinal difficulties, and dietary limitations.

During consultations with a certified dietician, patients may anticipate evidence-based dietary advice that is customized to their specific needs. This may include suggestions for meal planning, dish modification, quantity management, and supplements as required.

Furthermore, a licensed dietitian may assist patients in navigating contradictory information regarding nutrition and cancer that may be available online or elsewhere. They may give solid, science-based information to patients, allowing them to make more educated choices regarding their diet and general health.

Overall, receiving expert dietary counsel from a licensed dietitian may help cancer patients improve their quality of life, nutritional intake, and treatment results. Individuals who work with a skilled and supportive healthcare provider may better manage nutritional difficulties and optimize their well-being throughout the cancer journey.

# CHAPTER NINE

## Lifestyle Factors And Their Impact

## The Importance Of Exercise And Physical Activity

Exercise and physical exercise are critical for preserving overall health and well-being, particularly for testicular cancer patients. Regular exercise not only improves physical health but also promotes mental and emotional well-being.

Exercise may assist people with testicular cancer manage treatment adverse effects such as tiredness, nausea, and muscular weakness. It also helps to maintain a healthy body weight, which is critical for lowering the risk of cancer recurrence and enhancing treatment results.

When introducing exercise into your schedule, it's critical to begin softly and gradually increase the intensity and length of your exercises. This permits your body to adapt to the physical demands imposed on it, lowering the likelihood of damage.

Individuals with testicular cancer may benefit from a variety of workouts, including aerobic exercises like walking, cycling, and swimming, as well as strength training exercises to build muscular strength and endurance.

In addition to regular workouts, including physical activity in your everyday life might be advantageous. This might include things like walking the stairs instead of the lift, gardening, or playing sports with friends and family.

Individuals with testicular cancer may improve their general quality of life and their body's capacity to deal with treatment obstacles by prioritizing exercise and physical activity.

## Stress Management Techniques

Individuals receiving testicular cancer therapy must manage stress well. Chronic stress may damage the immune system, promote inflammation in the body, and impair treatment results. Thus, practicing appropriate stress management skills is critical for sustaining physical and emotional well-being throughout this difficult period.

Mindfulness meditation is an excellent stress-management method. Mindfulness is the practice of paying attention to the present moment without judgment, which may help to decrease anxiety and increase relaxation. Even only a few minutes of mindfulness meditation every day may help you manage stress effectively.

Deep breathing exercises are another effective stress-management approach. Deep breathing promotes the body's relaxation response, lowering stress hormone levels and generating a sensation of peace and relaxation. Taking calm, deep breaths and concentrating on the feeling of breathing may help reduce tension and anxiety.

Engaging in pleasant activities such as hobbies, spending time with loved ones, or listening to music may all help to decrease stress. It is important to prioritize self-care and schedule time for things that offer pleasure and relaxation.

In addition to these approaches, receiving assistance from friends, family, or a mental health professional may help you manage stress. Talking about your thoughts and worries with others may help you get emotional support and perspective, reducing stress and improving coping abilities.

Incorporating these stress management tactics into your daily routine can help you deal with the difficulties of testicular cancer treatment and enhance your overall quality of life.

# Quality Sleep And Its Role In Recovery

Quality sleep is critical for general health and well-being, especially for those being treated for testicular cancer. Adequate sleep helps the body repair and rejuvenate cells, strengthens the immune system, and promotes mental and emotional wellness.

Sleep disruptions are prevalent in cancer patients, including difficulties falling asleep, frequent waking throughout the night, and early morning awakenings. Sleep disruptions may be caused by a variety of circumstances, including discomfort, anxiety, drugs, and sleep pattern alterations.

To increase sleep quality, maintain a consistent sleep schedule and develop a soothing nighttime ritual. This might involve things like reading, having a warm bath, or practicing relaxation methods before bedtime. It is also beneficial to establish a good sleep environment, which includes a supportive mattress, comfy pillows, and a cool, dark, and quiet room.

Avoiding stimulants like coffee, nicotine, and electronic gadgets before bedtime may also help improve sleep quality. These medications may disrupt the body's normal sleep-wake cycle, making it more difficult to fall asleep.

If your sleep issues continue after these methods, speak with your healthcare physician. They may provide advice and help for managing sleep issues, such as suggesting drugs or treatments to enhance sleep quality.

Individuals with testicular cancer may improve their overall health and well-being by prioritizing quality sleep and practicing sleep hygiene methods that help the body's healing process.

# Avoiding Tobacco And Excessive Alcohol

Individuals receiving testicular cancer therapy should avoid smoking and drinking excessively. Tobacco use, including smoking and chewing tobacco, is known to increase the chance of developing numerous forms of cancer, including testicular cancer. Quitting smoking and avoiding tobacco products may help lower the chance of cancer recurrence and improve treatment results.

In addition to tobacco use, heavy alcohol use may hurt cancer therapy and recovery. Alcohol may impair the body's capacity to metabolize drugs, weaken the immune system, and raise the likelihood of problems during therapy.

Quitting smoking and limiting alcohol intake may be difficult, but there are tools and assistance available to help people achieve beneficial lifestyle choices.

Counseling, support groups, nicotine replacement treatment, and pharmaceuticals may all help people quit smoking.

Making lifestyle changes, such as quitting smoking and restricting alcohol intake, may have a major impact on testicular cancer patients' treatment results, reduce the chance of cancer recurrence, and improve general health and well-being.

## Social Support And Community Engagement

Individuals enduring testicular cancer treatment need strong social support and community involvement. A robust network of friends, family, and healthcare professionals may provide emotional support, practical aid, and encouragement throughout the treatment process.

Participating in discussions with people who have had similar experiences may also be useful. Support groups, both in-person and online, allow you to connect with others who understand what you're going through, exchange information and resources, and get encouragement and guidance.

In addition to official support groups, being connected with friends, family, and community organizations may give you a feeling of belonging and purpose at a difficult time. Volunteering, engaging in hobbies or recreational activities, and attending community events may all help people feel more connected to others while also maintaining a feeling of normality and regularity.

It is critical to explain your requirements and preferences to your support network, as well as how they can best help you during your cancer experience. Whether it's delivering physical assistance, listening ears, or just spending time together, social support is critical in helping people deal with the difficulties of testicular cancer treatment.

Individuals with testicular cancer who prioritize social support and community participation might feel supported, empowered, and more able to negotiate the ups and downs of their cancer experience.

# CHAPTER TEN

## Moving Forward: Long-Term Health And Wellness

## Importance Of Regular Follow-Up Care

Regular follow-up care is an important part of treating testicular cancer. After treatment, it is important to have a regular schedule of follow-up meetings with your healthcare professional. These consultations serve numerous reasons, including monitoring your healing progress, identifying any symptoms of recurrence early on, and dealing with any possible long-term therapy adverse effects.

During follow-up sessions, your healthcare team will do physical exams, blood tests, and imaging scans to evaluate your general health and look for symptoms of cancer recurrence.

These frequent checkups are critical for recognizing changes in your health quickly and providing appropriate action if necessary.

Furthermore, follow-up care allows you to share any concerns or questions you may have about your health or treatment with your healthcare professional. They can help you manage side effects, make lifestyle changes, and address any emotional or psychological issues you may be experiencing as a consequence of your cancer diagnosis and treatment.

Prioritizing frequent follow-up care allows you to actively monitor your health and achieve the best potential results in your long-term cancer journey.

## Monitoring For Recurrence And Secondary Cancers

One of the key purposes of follow-up care is to watch for indicators of cancer recurrence or the emergence of secondary malignancies.

Testicular cancer survivors are at risk of recurrence, especially in the first few years after therapy. Furthermore, several therapies, such as radiation therapy or chemotherapy, may raise the chance of acquiring additional malignancies later in life.

Your healthcare practitioner will do frequent physical examinations, imaging tests, and blood tests to detect recurrence and secondary malignancies. These tests aid in detecting any anomalies or changes that might suggest the existence of cancer. Early discovery is critical to successful treatment, thus keeping regular follow-up sessions is vital for efficiently monitoring your health condition.

It is critical that you be watchful and quickly report any new symptoms or concerns to your healthcare physician. By being proactive and involved in your follow-up care, you may collaborate with your healthcare team to identify and treat any possible cancer-related complications early on.

# Healthy Lifestyle As A Preventive Measure

Maintaining a healthy lifestyle is critical for avoiding cancer recurrence and improving general well-being after treatment. Adopting healthy behaviors may help lower the chance of cancer recurrence, improve treatment results, and improve the overall quality of life.

A well-balanced diet high in fruits, vegetables, whole grains, and lean meats contains critical nutrients that promote immune function and general health. Avoiding excessive alcohol intake, tobacco use, and processed meals rich in sugar and harmful fats may also help to avoid cancer.

Regular physical exercise is another essential component of a healthy lifestyle. Regular exercise not only helps to maintain a healthy weight, but it also lowers the risk of chronic illnesses and boosts mood and vitality.

In addition to food and exercise, controlling stress and prioritizing mental health are critical components of total well-being. Mindfulness, meditation, and relaxation practices may help decrease stress and improve emotional well-being.

By taking a holistic approach to health and wellbeing, you may help your body's natural capacity to recover and flourish after cancer treatment.

## Advocacy And Raising Awareness

Advocacy and increasing awareness are critical in assisting persons impacted by testicular cancer and encouraging early identification and treatment. As a survivor, you may be an effective advocate for yourself and others by telling your experience, raising awareness about the significance of early diagnosis, and pushing for access to excellent treatment and services.

Participating in community events, fundraising activities, and awareness campaigns may help people learn about testicular cancer, debunk myths and misunderstandings, and promote proactive health habits. By speaking out and contributing to the cause, you can make a significant difference in the lives of individuals affected by this illness.

Furthermore, pushing for laws and programs that promote cancer research, prevention, and patient support services may help improve outcomes for people suffering from testicular cancer and other forms of cancer.

You can help cancer survivors have a better future by advocating and spreading awareness, as well as empowering others to take responsibility for their health and well-being.

# Resources For Ongoing Support And Information

Access to continuing care and information is critical for testicular cancer patients and their loved ones. Fortunately, several organizations, support groups, and online communities exist to provide information, aid, and encouragement throughout the cancer experience.

These sites include a variety of services, including instructional materials, peer support programs, counseling services, and practical aid in navigating healthcare systems and finding treatment alternatives. Whether you're looking for information on treatment side effects, coping tactics, or financial assistance, there are options available to match your requirements.

In addition to professional support programs, socializing with other cancer survivors and carers may offer vital emotional support and motivation. Sharing your experiences, views, and suggestions with those who have been down the same road may help you feel more connected and empowered.

You may establish a strong network of allies and resources to assist you in negotiating the obstacles of life after testicular cancer by making use of available services and seeking help when required.

# CONCLUSION

To summarise, although the association between food and testicular cancer is complicated and diverse, there is evidence that specific dietary components may increase or decrease the chance of acquiring this kind of cancer.

According to studies, eating a diet rich in fruits, vegetables, and whole grains, as well as avoiding processed meats and saturated fats, may reduce the risk of testicular cancer. Furthermore, keeping a healthy weight and engaging in regular physical exercise may help to reduce the risk of having this condition.

However, it is critical to recognize the limits of existing research, since many studies on nutrition and testicular cancer are based on self-reported data and retrospective analysis, which may introduce bias and mistakes.

Furthermore, individual genetic predispositions and environmental variables impact cancer risk, making it difficult to establish a clear link between certain food components and testicular cancer.

As a result, although a balanced and nutritious diet combined with a healthy lifestyle may have potential advantages in lowering the incidence of testicular cancer, further study is required to better understand the underlying processes and create more effective preventative techniques. Furthermore, early diagnosis via frequent self-examinations and medical tests is critical in improving outcomes for those who are at risk of or have been diagnosed with testicular cancer.

**THE END**

Made in the USA
Columbia, SC
12 March 2025